SOTHIS PRESS

Sothis Press aims to completely reimagine the public domain book with an emphasis on universal access to captivatingly designed print editions. We believe that technology will enable every single book ever published to be perpetually accessible in beautiful print form. Sothis is beauty in ubiquity.

www.sothis.press
1 Waterhouse Square, London, ECIN 2ST

The Hygienic System, or the Principles of Hygienic Medication Briefly Explained

A Work for Inquiries

E. T. Robinson

SOTHIS PRESS

ISBN 978-1-0365-1718-2

The Hygienic System, or the Principles of Hygienic Medication Briefly Explained is in the public domain.

THE HYGIENIC SYSTEM.

BY

E. T. ROBINSON, M. D.,
A GRADUATE OF THE NEW YORK HYGEIO THERAPEUTIC COLLEGE.

POMFRET, CT.
PUBLISHED BY E. T. ROBINSON.
1870.

THE

HYGIENIC SYSTEM:

OR

THE PRINCIPLES OF HYGIENIC MEDICATION BRIEFLY EXPLAINED.

A WORK FOR INQUIRERS,

BY E. T. ROBINSON, M. D.,
A GRADUATE OF THE NEW YORK HYGEIO-THERAPEUTIC COLLEGE.

POMFRET, CT.
PUBLISHED BY E. T. ROBINSON.
1870.

SNOW BROS., PRS., WORCESTER, MASS.

INTRODUCTION.

It is not the design of this little book to discuss the details of the Hygienic System, but simply to give a brief explanation of some of its leading principles, and put them in a cheap form, so as to be within the reach of all. To those who wish to pursue the inquiry further, the author would recommend Dr. Trall's "Hydropathic Encyclopedia," also, Dr. Jackson's "How to Treat the Sick without Medicine." There are also several good journals published, of which "The Health Reformer," and "The Laws of Life," are the best.

The author knows that there are large numbers of sick persons in all parts of the world, suffering from disease without hope of relief, who, if they could be made acquainted with this system, would seek relief and find it, without doubt. For such, this work is especially designed. The author would also invite the attention of Philanthropists and Christians to a system which discards *alcohol* as a remedial agent, and all other things which tend to arouse human passions and excite the propensities arise, to the doctrine here taught, in the minds of of man. He is aware that many objections will those who have not investigated this subject; but the reader is assured that the objections can all be answered, the only regret is that the limits of this tract will not permit the discussion. There is much that goes in the world by the name of Hygiene, but the true system is the result of experience in the application of Hygienic agencies to the treatment of the sick, as well as to the maintainence of health in those who are well.

The author acknowledges his obligations to Prof. Trall, to whom the world is indebted for the solution of many problems pertaining to the Healing Art. He would also thank the Professors of the H. T. College, to whom he is indebted for much valuable information.

The paragraphs in italics are in the language of Prof. R. T. Trall, and were taken from *The Catalogue of the Hygeio-Therapeutic College.*

THE HYGIENIC SYSTEM.

1. "*All healing power is inherent in the living System.*"

That the human body has the power to recover, under favorable circumstances, from most of the injuries that may be inflicted upon it, no observing person will pretend to deny. For instance: if a person cuts his flesh or breaks a bone, place the part under favorable conditions and the healing power of nature which resides in the part injured will restore it again, in a short time, to its former state of health. Again, if a person takes cold or injures himself by over-work, a little care, or rest for a time, will allow nature to recuperate and restore the body to health. So of other diseases and injuries to which a person may be exposed. Only give nature a fair chance and she will always prove herself able to right the wrongs that may be inflicted upon her.

The existence of such a healing power in

the human body has been recognized by medical men in all ages of the world. Some of the ablest minds of the profession have frequently acknowledged and proclaimed this fact. That this power exists in the living system alone, and nowhere else, I shall endeavor to prove.

2. "*There is no curative 'virtue' in medicines, nor in anything outside the vital organism.*"

This proposition is contrary to the almost universal belief of mankind. It is nevertheless true, and proven by the following facts: In the first place the world is full of invalids or persons who are partially crippled in some one or more of their powers. Indeed it is a rare thing to find a person who is perfectly sound in health of body or vigor of mind, and so accustomed have people become to sickness and disease that no one considers himself sick unless he is confined to his bed. Those who are able to keep about and attend to business are considered perfectly healthy, yet there are very few who have not some chronic disease. Yet the world is full of "medicine," and there are at least 50,000 physicians in the United States alone. It is not necessary to consult the newspapers to learn the number of patent medicines in vogue, each of which is warranted to cure (?) certain diseases. Millions of dollars are annually expended in advertising these nostrums, and princely fortunes are amassed in the traffic; yet few persons claim to have been cured by them.

It is true that many persons who have *acute* diseases, (those of short continuance) recover. They take medicine and the recovery is attributed to that. Nature does the work and the medicine gets the credit. They would get well under almost any circumstances; yet thousands annually die of diseases that are not intrinsically dangerous. They die in consequence of wrong treatment, and many wonderful cures are fortunate escapes. Thousands recover from acute diseases and have terrible forms of chronic diseases, (those of long continuance) in consequence. These are are the results of the *drugs* that have been administered. Such results are never known in Hygienic Practice.

Our proposition is further proven by the fact that the older physicians grow the less faith they have in the power of medicine, and the more in nature to cure disease. And those who give the least medicine and attend more to the Hygienic condition of their patients, are the most successful in their practice.

Again, the practice of Hygienic Physicians, who do not use medicine at all, but rely wholly upon Hygienic agencies, bears still stronger evidence. They rarely lose a case of acute disease, and succeed in curing 90 per cent. of the chronic cases that come to them. All may be benefitted or made more comfortable.

The popular belief in the curative powers of medicine amounts to a superstition. It is unworthy of the enlightenment of the nineteenth century. It is a relic of the dark ages, when charms and incantations were the means resorted to, to cure the sick.

3. '*Nature has not provided remedies for diseases.*'

Although this statement is absolutely true, it needs a little explanation on account of the popular belief to the contrary. Every phenomenon in nature has a *cause*; this is true of disease. Disease is the effect of a cause, is in short the *penalty* of the violation of nature's *laws*. Nature has provided penalties then for the violation of her laws; how then can it be supposed that she has provided remedies to do away with the penalties? Such a supposition would be absurd. Suppose our legislature should establish a penalty for theft, and then say if the culprit will only take a bottle of "Plantation Bitters" the penalty will be removed? "No!" they say "serve out your time and then return to obedience." So says nature: "Obey my laws and live;" "Return to obedience and I will forgive." The *healing power* being already *in the living system*, why should we look further?

4. "*There is no "law of cure" in the universe; and the only condition of cure is, obedience to physiological law.*"

By "law of cure" is meant the "*contraria*

contrarius curantur," (unlike cures unlike) of the allopathists, and the "*similia similibus curantur*," (like cures like) of the homœopathists. The absurd supposition that one disease can cure another! What becomes of the patient meantime? The truth of this proposition follows from what we have already said, that cures depend upon the *condition of obedience*.*

5. "*Remedial agents do not act upon the living system, as is taught in medical books and schools, but are acted on by the vital powers.*"

This follows from a law of nature which is universal, to-wit: The relation of living and dead matter—"*living matter is active and dead matter passive*"—when they come in contact with each other. By living matter is meant anything that has life, and dead matter anything that has not life. When a poisonous substance is taken into the system, the vital powers set to work to resist it and to expel it. Every organ it comes in contact with sets up a defensive struggle. This is vital resistance; it is disease. The same thing happens when obstructions occur in the body by matter retained which should be expelled. If food be taken it is transformed into the tissues of the body. This is physiological action; it is *health*.

---

*NOTE.—Disease being a "remedial effort," is often successful under unfavorable circumstances, hence the patient gets well; but "remedial efforts" are not always successful, hence the need of a physician to assist nature by supplying favorable conditions.

6. "*Disease is not, as is supposed, an enemy at war with the vital powers, but a remedial effort, a process of purification and reparation. It is not a thing to be destroyed, subdued or suppressed, but an action to be regulated and directed.*"

Disease then is an *action* on the part of the living system—a "Remedial Effort;" not indeed an effort to remedy another disease, but to remove obstructions and repair damages. This follows from what we have said under 1 and 5. This may be illustrated by cholera, in which the vomiting and purging, &c., are efforts on the part of the system to rid itself of impurities.

7. "*True remedial agents are materials and influences which have normal relations to the vital organs, and not drugs or poisons, whose relations are abnormal and anti-vital.*"

By "normal" agents is meant those that were intended by nature to be used, and by "abnormal" is meant those that are unnatural and consequently injurious. It is true that medicines will often alleviate *pain*, and so far they may be useful when people do not know any better way. But *pain* is not disease; it is only the voice of nature crying out for help. It is one thing to silence the out-cries of nature for assistance, but quite another to remove the cause which occasions all the trouble.

8. "*Nature's Materia Medica, (medical material) consists of air, light, heat, electricity, magnetism, exercise, rest, food, drink, bathing, sleep, clothing, passional influences, and mechanical or surgical appliances.*"

People get sick by the misuse of these things as well as by the use of things abnormal or unnatural. In all their relations of life they disobey the laws of health, chiefly through ignorance. They make bad selections of food; they eat many things that are not food, and that which is good they spoil by a vitiated system of cookery and their appetites have become perverted and unnatural. Many breathe impure air, over-work and neglect cleanliness; thus they become sick, and then to make a bad matter worse they rush for a medicine bottle, and thus chronic diseases are fastened upon them. People thus debilitated are unable to endure the vicissitudes of weather and climate as well as the changes of season to which it falls to the lot of most people to be exposed, and they become an easy prey to the arch-destroyer, DEATH.

9. "*The True Healing Art, consists in supplying the living system with whatever of the above materials it can use under the circumstances, and not in the adminstration of poisons which it must Resist and Expel.*

In the Hygienic agencies mentioned we have ample resources for the treatment of every disease "that flesh is heir to." By adapting them to the condition of the patient we can cure every curable person, and render all more comfortable. With the simple agent WATER, with the assistance of certain instruments and appliances, we can remove all obstructions, and that too without any injury to the patient. In the treatment of inflammations and congestions there is no more efficient agent than WATER, and in skillful hands there never need be any injury from its use.

One great advantage in our treatment consists in taking away the bad things and supplying those that are good. We assist NATURE in the truest sense of the word. Drugs, on the contrary, only hinder nature's efforts; they suppress the action constituting disease, but do not cure the patient; THAT is always the work of nature, if it is done at all.

10. "*Drugs are themselves causes of disease. If they remove one disease it is only by produceing a drug disease. Every dose diminishes the vitality of the patient.*"

This statement is proven by the fact, that if a course of "medicine," which would be given by an allopathic physician in the treatment of any disease, were given to a well person it would make him sick. This is shown in the homœopathic "provings." The Homœopathists take a well person and give him a drug in anallopathic dose, and note its effect; this shows its nature. This is then diluted or attenuated and given in minute quantities on the principle of "SIMILIA, &C." "Every dose diminishes the vitality of the patient," because it requires an exertion of life power to expel it. The vitality is the sum total of a person's life force, and as every one has a certain FUND OF LIFE FORCE which cannot be increased, every particle expended uselessly is so much wasted. "Vitality once lost can never be regained." The injury done by "medicine" is proportional to the quantity taken.

11. "*Drugopathy endeavors to restore health by administering the poisons which produce disease.*"

This is done under an erroneous idea of the nature of disease and of the relation of remedies to the living system.

12. "*Hygeio-Therapy (Hygienic Medication), erroneously called "Hydropathy" or "Water Cure," on the contrary, restores the sick to health by the means which preserves health in well persons.*"

It removes the cause of disease and supplies nature with the means for recovery.

13. "*Diseases are caused by obstructions, the obstructing materials being poisons or impurities of some kind.*"

The truth of this follows from what has already been said.

14. "*The Hygienic System removes these obstructions and leaves the body sound.*"

This is the true way to treat disease.

15. "*Drug medicines add to the causes of obstructions and change acute into chronic diseases.*"

Chronic diseases are characterized by deficient vitality. When drugs "cure" (?) disease, it is by exciting nature to increased effort, and thereby exhausting the vitality of the patient and consequently leaving him with debilitated organs. Hygienic Medication cures disease without the unnecessary exhaustion of the patient's vitality. When a patient recovers from a disease under drug treatment he usually is a long time convalescing. When a person recovers under Hygienic treatment he goes about his business as well as ever.

16. "*To attempt to cure disease by adding to the causes of disease, is irrational and absurd.*"

Does it not strike you so, Reader? If people were not ignorant of the real nature of medicine they would discard the whole drug system at once.

The Hygienic System not only teaches how to cure disease, but also how to avoid being sick, and it does more than that, for its universal adoption would tend to do away with vice and crime, and thereby add to the sum total of human happiness.

17. "*Hygienic Medication is not a one-ideaism which professes to cure all diseases, with "water alone;" nor is it a "Cold Water Cure," as is erroneously believed by many. It adopts all the remedial appliances in existence, with the single exception of* POISONS."

The Hygienic System is not an impracticable theory which seems very fine to read about; but it is a SYSTEM which is the product of many minds, founded in sound philosophy, and sustained by the experience of thousands of persons, and has been tested for more than a quarter of a century. Its philosophy of living has been adopted by more than 100,000 persons and it is gaining in popularity every day.

THE END.

Spotted something that isn't quite right?

Let us know and we'll fix it for future reprints. And as a thank you for your diligence, we'll send you a free Sothis book of your choice.

publisher@sothis.press

This page intentionally left blank

Except of course for that line above. And this one.
And whilst we have your attention, perhaps you'd
like to follow us on Instagram @sothis.press. Go on.

Made in United States
Orlando, FL
04 November 2026

90201511R00018